Love Knows No Age:

Finding Passion

In Your 60s And Beyond

Ingrid-Astrid Von Anhalt

Disclaimer

The advice and guidance provided in this publication are intended for general informational purposes only. The author and publisher make no representations or warranties of any kind, express or implied, about the completeness, accuracy, reliability, suitability, or availability of the content contained herein.

Any reliance you place on such information is strictly at your own risk. The author and publisher disclaim any liability for any loss or damage, including, without limitation, indirect or consequential loss or damage, or any loss or damage whatsoever arising from reliance on the advice and guidance provided in this publication.

Furthermore, the advice and guidance provided in this publication may not be intended for implementing any recommendations. The views and opinions expressed in this publication are those of the individual, organization, or entity.

This disclaimer applies to the fullest extent permitted by applicable law and shall survive any termination or expiration of this publication.

Table of Contents

Dedication

I dedicate this book to those who steadfastly believe in the transformative power of love, and to seekers of the enduring beauty and resilience of love that is possible.

May this book inspire you, when searching to embrace love with open arms, to have faith that every endeavor is worthwhile, with the undying hope and beauty found within the human heart.

Acknowledgment

I am deeply grateful to those individuals whose unwavering support, encouragement, and inspiration have been instrumental in the creation of this guide.

I thank all those whose honesty has touched my heart and motivated me to write. Thank you to my friends for their encouragement, and I thank God for making me recognize that helping others is one's duty in life and for reminding me of the power of words.

About the Author

Ingrid-Astrid is an Australian author whose work delves into various layers of culture and the ever-evolving landscape of relationships. With a passion for writing, she creates uplifting and often provocative content that challenges social norms and invites readers to think differently about love, identity, age, power, and belonging.

She is particularly interested in disrupting conventional thinking and inspiring meaningful reflection, encouraging her readers to question the status quo and embrace a different perspective on life. After a successful career in the commercial sector, she has exchanged the boardroom for a more expressive life, where her commitment to new approaches continues to thrive.

Introduction

In the quiet corners of our lives, where the echoes of youthful passions may have faded, a different kind of love can blossom. This book is a testament to the enduring power of love: love that knows no age, no boundaries, and no limits. It is a celebration of the wisdom and experience that come with growing older, and the unique beauty of finding passion in our 60s and beyond.

Throughout the pages ahead, we will explore what it means to navigate the landscape of love later in life. This journey is not just about romantic relationships; it is about self-discovery, resilience, and the profound connections that enrich our lives. It is a journey that many of us embark on with trepidation, yet with an unwavering hope for companionship, understanding, and deep emotional fulfillment.

In these chapters, you will find practical guidance and heartfelt reflections on building meaningful relationships at this stage of life. We will delve into the nuances of dating, communication, and intimacy, offering insights gathered from real experiences and expert advice. Whether you are starting anew, navigating the complexities of widowhood, or embracing the joys of companionship after a long journey alone, this book is here to support you.

Through stories, anecdotes, and practical tips, we aim to inspire and empower you on your quest for love. Each chapter is crafted with care and empathy, recognizing the unique challenges and joys that come with seeking and nurturing love later in life. Our goal is to illuminate the path ahead, offering reassurance and encouragement as you explore the possibilities that lie before you.

As you turn the pages, remember that you are not alone on this journey. Many have walked this path before you, and their stories of resilience and discovery light the way. Embrace the adventure of love in your 60s and beyond. It is a journey filled with hope, renewal, and the promise of a love that grows richer with each passing day.

Thank you for joining us on this exploration of love and possibility. May these words serve as a beacon of hope and guidance as you embark on this deeply rewarding chapter of your life.

Chapter: 01

Embracing Love and Passion at Any Age

Redefining Love and Passion in Your 60s

One of the key aspects of redefining love and passion in your 60s is letting go of societal expectations and embracing your authentic self. This is a time to be true to who you are and what you want out of life. It is a time to prioritize your own happiness and well-being rather than trying to please others.

In your 60s, love and passion take on a new depth and meaning. It is about creating connections that are based on mutual respect, understanding, and shared values. It is about nurturing relationships that bring out the best in you and your partner and supporting each other through life's ups and downs.

Embracing love and passion in your 60s also means being open to new experiences and adventures. It is about trying new things, stepping out of your comfort zone, and embracing the unknown. Whether it is traveling to a new destination, taking up a new hobby, or simply spending quality time with loved ones, there are endless opportunities to find joy and fulfillment in this stage of life.

In conclusion, love knows no age. By challenging stereotypes, surrounding yourself with supportive individuals, and communicating openly with your partner, you can overcome age stereotypes in relationships and find passion and fulfillment in your

60s and beyond. Embrace your age and all the possibilities that come with it and remember that love is timeless.

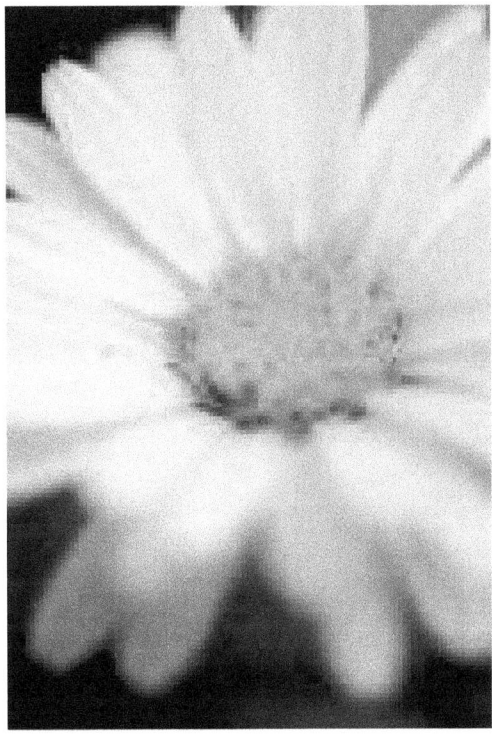

Overcoming Age Stereotypes in Relationships

As people age, they often face stereotypes and misconceptions about love and relationships. One common stereotype is that as we get older, we lose touch, lose desire, and lose passion and intimacy. However, the truth is that love knows no age. In fact, many people over 60 are finding new and exciting ways to experience love and passion in their later years.

To overcome age stereotypes in relationships, it is important to first challenge these beliefs within ourselves. Remember that age is just a number, and there is no expiration date on love or passion. Embrace your age and all the wisdom and experience that come with it.

Another key to overcoming age stereotypes in relationships is to surround yourself with supportive and open-minded individuals. Seek out friends and partners who value and respect you for who you are, regardless of your age. Surrounding yourself with positive influences can help you feel more confident and empowered in your relationships.

It is also important to communicate openly and honestly with your partner about your desires and needs. Do not be afraid to express your feelings and listen actively to your partner's needs as well. By fostering open and honest communication, you can build a stronger and more fulfilling relationship regardless of your age.

As we age, our definition of love and passion evolves. In our 60s and beyond, we have the opportunity to redefine what love and passion mean to us. It is a time to explore new possibilities, embrace change, and discover what truly brings us joy and fulfillment.

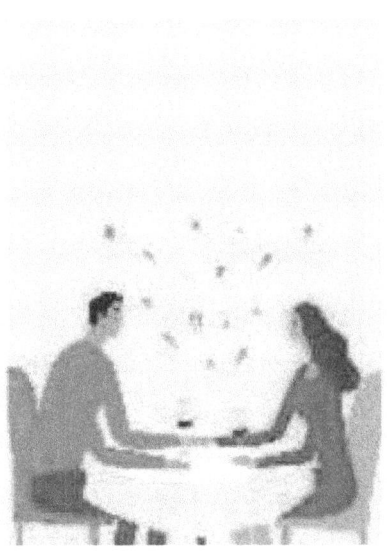

Exploring New Ways to Express Love and Passion

As we age, it is essential to continue exploring new ways to express love and passion in our lives. In our 60s and beyond, we may find that the conventional ways of showing love no longer resonate with us. This is the perfect time to get creative and think outside the box when it comes to expressing our feelings for our partners.

One way to explore new ways to express love and passion is through acts of kindness and thoughtfulness. Small gestures, such as leaving love notes around the house or surprising your partner with their favorite meal, can go a long way in showing your love and affection. These simple acts can reignite the spark in your relationship and remind your partner how much you care.

Another way to express love and passion in your 60s and beyond is through physical touch. Holding hands, cuddling, and even dancing together can strengthen the bond between you and your partner. Physical touch is a powerful way to communicate your love and affection, and it can help you feel more connected to your partner on a deeper level.

Exploring new ways to express love and passion can also involve trying new activities together. Whether it is taking a dance class, going on a romantic getaway, or learning a new hobby, sharing new experiences can bring you closer and reignite the passion in your relationship. By stepping out of your comfort zone and trying new things together, you can create lasting memories and strengthen your bond.

Exploring new ways to express love and passion in your 60s and beyond can help you keep the flame alive in your relationship. By being creative, thoughtful, and adventurous, you can show your partner how much you love them in unique and meaningful ways. Love truly knows no age, and it is never too late to find passion in your relationship.

Chapter 02:

Rediscovering Yourself in Your 60s

Embracing Self-Confidence and Self-Love

In your 60s and beyond, it is more important than ever to embrace self-confidence and self-love. This is the time in your life when you have gained wisdom and experience, and it is crucial to recognize your worth and value. By practicing self-confidence and self-love, you can truly embrace the beauty of aging and find a renewed passion for life.

Self-confidence is about believing in yourself and in your abilities. It is about knowing that you are capable of achieving your goals and dreams, no matter your age. Take the time to reflect on your past accomplishments and successes and use them as a source of inspiration to move forward. Surround yourself with positive influences and remind yourself daily of your strengths and capabilities.

Self-love goes hand in hand with self-confidence. It is about accepting yourself fully, flaws and all, and treating yourself with kindness and compassion. Take the time to practice self-care and prioritize your physical, mental, and emotional well-being. This could be through activities like meditation, exercise, or spending time with loved ones who uplift you.

By embracing self-confidence and self-love, you can cultivate a deeper sense of love and passion in your relationships. When you love and value yourself, you can more easily give and receive love from others. This can lead to more fulfilling and meaningful connections with your partner, friends, and family members. Remember, age is just a number, and it is never too late to embrace self-confidence and self-love. By doing so, you can find a renewed sense of passion and purpose in your 60s and beyond. Embrace your worth and value and let your light shine brightly for all to see.

In conclusion, do not be afraid to pursue your hobbies and interests with enthusiasm. Embrace the things that bring you joy and let them enrich your life in ways you never thought possible. Love knows no age, and neither does passion.

Pursuing Hobbies And Interest That Bring You Joy

Love knows no age, and neither does passion, so go out there and find what truly makes your soul come alive.

As we enter our 60s and beyond, it is more important than ever to prioritize activities that bring us joy and fulfillment. One of the best ways to do this is by pursuing hobbies and interests that we are truly passionate about.

Many of us may have spent years focusing on our careers, raising a family, or taking care of others, often putting our own interests on the back burner. Now is the time to rediscover those passions and delve into activities that bring us happiness.

Whether it is painting, gardening, playing an instrument, or trying out a new sport, engaging in hobbies can have numerous benefits for our overall well-being. Not only do they provide a sense of accomplishment and purpose, but they also help to reduce stress and improve mental clarity. Furthermore, pursuing hobbies can be a great way to meet new people and expand our social circles. Joining a club or group related to our interests can lead to meaningful connections and friendships, fostering a sense of community and belonging.

By actively seeking out activities that bring us joy, we are able to cultivate a sense of fulfillment and satisfaction in our lives. It is never too late to explore new interests and passions, so why not take the time to indulge in activities that make your heart sing.

Reflecting on Past Relationships and Lessons Learned

As we reach our 60s and beyond, it is natural to reflect on our past relationships and the lessons we have learned along the way. These experiences have shaped us into the individuals we are today and have paved the way for us to find love and passion in our later years.

Reflecting on past relationships can be a powerful way to gain insight into what we truly want and need in a partner. It is an opportunity to examine the dynamics of our past relationships, what worked well, and what did not. By looking back on these experiences, we can identify patterns and behaviors that may have hindered our ability to find lasting love and passion.

One important lesson that many of us learn from past relationships is the importance of communication and compromise. These are essential components of any successful relationship, and without them, it can be challenging to build a strong and lasting connection with a partner. By reflecting on past relationships, we can learn how to better communicate our needs and desires and how to work together with our partner to find solutions to conflicts and challenges.

Another valuable lesson we can learn from past relationships is the importance of self-love and self-care. It is essential to prioritize our own well-being and happiness in a relationship, as this sets the foundation for a healthy and fulfilling partnership. By reflecting on past relationships, we can identify times when we may have neglected our own needs and learn how to prioritize self-love in future relationships.

Overall, reflecting on past relationships can provide us with valuable insights and lessons that can help us find love and passion in our 60s and beyond. By learning from our past experiences, we can build stronger and more fulfilling relationships moving forward.

Chapter 03:

Navigating Dating and Relationships in Your 60s

Embracing Online Dating and Meeting New People

In today's digital age, online dating has become a popular way for people over 60 to meet new potential partners and explore romantic relationships. Embracing online dating can open up a whole new world of opportunities for those looking to find love and passion in their 60s and beyond.

One of the key benefits of online dating for people over 60 is the ability to connect with a wider range of individuals who share similar interests and values. This can be especially helpful for those who may not have as many opportunities to meet new people in their day-to-day lives. By creating a profile on a dating site or app, you can easily browse through potential matches and start conversations with those who catch your eye.

Online dating also allows you to take things at your own pace and get to know someone before meeting in person. This can help alleviate any anxieties or uncertainties you may have about dating again later in life. Additionally, many dating platforms offer features such as video calls and messaging, which can help you build a connection with someone before taking the next step to meet face-to-face.

Meeting new people through online dating can be a fun and exciting experience, and it is never too late to find love and passion in your 60s and beyond. Do not be afraid to create a profile, upload a recent photo, and start exploring the possibilities that online dating has to offer. You never know—your perfect match could be just a click away.

As we age, our priorities and desires in relationships may shift, but one thing remains constant: the need for trust and intimacy. Building trust and intimacy in later relationships can be a rewarding experience that deepens the connection between partners and creates a strong foundation for love and passion to flourish.

Building Trust and Intimacy in Later Relationships

Intimacy in later relationships is not just about physical closeness; it is also about emotional and spiritual connection. Take the time to truly get to know your partner on a deeper level, exploring their likes, dislikes, dreams, and fears. Share meaningful experiences together, whether it is trying new activities, traveling to new places, or simply spending quality time together at home.

Another important aspect of building trust and intimacy in later relationships is forgiveness. As we age, we may carry baggage from past relationships or experiences that can impact our current partnership. Learning to forgive and let go of past hurts can help you move forward together and create a stronger bond.

Be honest with your partner about your needs and desires, both in and out of the bedroom. Discuss what brings you joy and fulfillment and explore new ways to connect and express your love. By being open and transparent about your wants and needs, you can create a more satisfying and passionate relationship.

Remember, building trust and intimacy in later relationships takes time and effort. Be patient with each other, communicate openly and honestly, and make an effort to nurture your connection every day. By prioritizing trust and intimacy, you can create a lasting and fulfilling relationship that brings joy and passion well into your 60s and beyond.

As we age, our bodies and desires may change, but that does not mean physical intimacy and sexual health should be neglected. In fact, embracing these aspects of our lives can lead to a renewed sense of passion and connection in our 60s and beyond.

Communicating Openly and Honestly with Your Partner

One of the keys to building trust in a later relationship is open and honest communication. It is important to share your thoughts, feelings, and fears with your partner, as well as to listen actively to their concerns. By being vulnerable and transparent with each other, you can create a safe space where trust can grow.

Successful communication involves active listening. Truly listen to your partner without interrupting or judging. Show empathy and understanding and validate their feelings. By creating a safe space for open dialogue, you can foster trust and intimacy in your relationship.

Communication is key in any relationship, but it becomes even more crucial as we age and our needs and desires evolve. As we grow older, we may face new challenges and experiences that can impact our relationships. It is essential to have open and honest conversations with your partner about your feelings, fears, and desires. By sharing your thoughts and emotions, you can strengthen your bond and ensure that both partners feel heard and understood. Be receptive to their feedback. By working together to communicate openly and honestly, you can navigate the ups and downs of aging with grace and compassion.

By talking openly about your needs and desires, you can ensure that both you and your partner are on the same page when it comes to keeping your relationship exciting and maintaining a strong and passionate connection in your 60s and beyond.

In conclusion, while relationships may change as we age, there are always new ways to keep the passion alive. By trying new things together, prioritizing intimacy, and communicating openly, you can ensure that your relationship remains exciting and fulfilling for years to come. Love knows no age, and with a little effort, you can keep the flame of passion burning bright in your relationship, no matter how old you are.

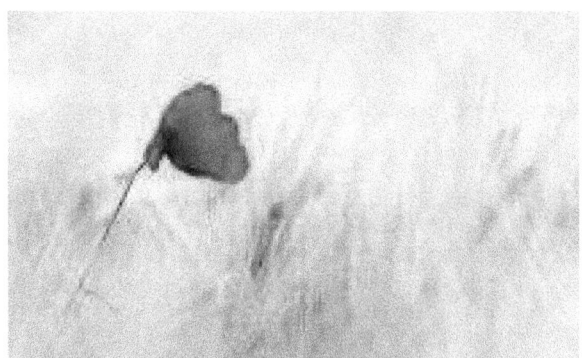

Chapter 04:

Keeping the Spark Alive in Your 60s and Beyond

Exploring New Ways to Keep Your Relationship Exciting

As we age, it can be easy for relationships to fall into a routine and lose some of their excitement. However, it is important to remember that love knows no age, and there are always new ways to keep the passion alive in your relationship, no matter how long you have been together.

One way to keep your relationship exciting is to try new things together. Whether it is taking up a new hobby, exploring a new city, or trying a new restaurant, stepping out of your comfort zone can reignite the spark in your relationship. By sharing new experiences, you can create lasting memories and deepen your bond with your partner.

Another way to keep your relationship exciting is to prioritize intimacy. Physical touch and affection are important components of a healthy relationship, so make sure to set aside time for romance and intimacy. Whether it is through cuddling, holding hands, or trying new things in the bedroom, keeping the physical aspect of your relationship alive can help keep the passion burning bright.

Physical intimacy is an important part of any relationship, regardless of age. It can help us feel closer to our partners, reduce stress, and even improve our overall health. As we age, it is important to communicate openly with our partners about our needs and desires. This can help ensure that both partners feel satisfied and valued in their relationship.

When it comes to sexual health, many people over 60 may have concerns or questions. It is important to remember that sexual health is an integral part of overall wellness. Taking care of our sexual health should include regular checkups with healthcare providers, practicing safe sex, and exploring new ways to connect with our partners.

Embracing Physical Intimacy and Sexual Health

For those who may be experiencing changes in their sexual health, such as erectile dysfunction or menopause, it is essential to seek support and guidance from healthcare professionals. There are many treatment options available that can help improve sexual function and satisfaction.

Ultimately, embracing physical intimacy and sexual health in our 60s and beyond can lead to a more fulfilling and vibrant life. By prioritizing these aspects of our relationships, we can nurture our connection with our partners and continue to experience love and passion at any age. Love truly knows no age, and with an open mind and heart, we can continue to find joy and fulfillment in our relationships.

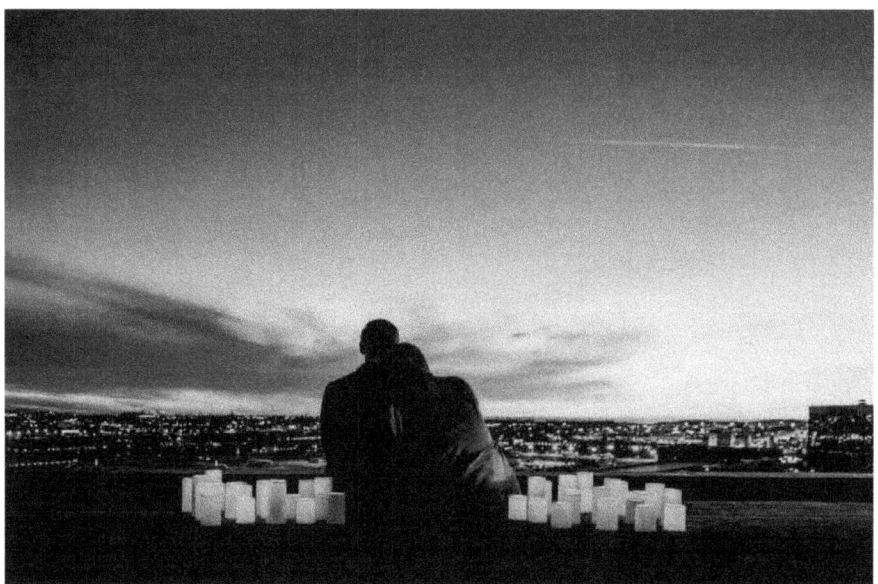

Cultivating Emotional Intimacy and Connection with Your Partner

One of the most fulfilling aspects of being in a loving relationship is the emotional intimacy and connection you share with your partner. As we age, it becomes even more crucial to nurture and cultivate these aspects of our relationships. In our 60s and beyond, we have the wisdom and experience to truly appreciate the value of emotional intimacy and connection.

To foster emotional intimacy with your partner, it is important to communicate openly and honestly. Share your thoughts, feelings, and fears with each other. Be vulnerable and allow yourself to be truly seen by your partner. This level of honesty and vulnerability can deepen your emotional connection and strengthen your bond.

Another way to cultivate emotional intimacy is to show empathy and understanding toward your partner. Listen actively and attentively when they speak and try to see things from their perspective. Empathy is a powerful tool for building emotional intimacy and creating a sense of closeness with your partner.

In addition to communication and empathy, spending quality time together is essential for maintaining emotional intimacy. Whether it is going for a walk, cooking a meal together, or simply cuddling on the couch, find activities that you both enjoy and make time for them regularly. This shared time will help you feel more connected and emotionally attuned to each other.

By prioritizing emotional intimacy and connection in your relationship, you can enjoy a deeper, more fulfilling partnership in your 60s and beyond. Remember that love knows no age, and with effort and dedication, you can continue to find passion and joy in your relationship for years to come.

Chapter 05:

Overcoming Challenges and

Celebrating Victories

Dealing with Age-Related Health Issues in Relationships

As we age, it is natural for our bodies to undergo changes that can affect our health and well-being. In relationships, these age-related health issues can present unique challenges that require understanding, patience, and open communication.

One of the most common age-related health issues that couples may face is decreased energy levels. As we get older, our bodies may not have the same stamina and vitality that they once did. This can impact on our ability to engage in physical activities with our partners, such as going for long walks or participating in sports. It is important for couples to be honest with each other about their energy levels and to find activities they can enjoy together at a pace that is comfortable for both partners.

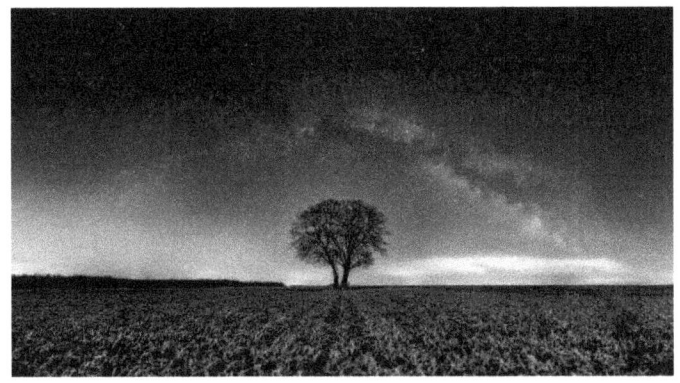

Another age-related health issue that can affect relationships is chronic pain. Many people over 50 experience conditions such as arthritis or back pain that can make it difficult to engage in physical intimacy. It is crucial for partners to communicate openly about any pain or discomfort they may be experiencing and to explore alternative ways of connecting and expressing their love for each other.

Additionally, as we age, our bodies may be more susceptible to certain health conditions, such as heart disease or diabetes. It is important for couples to support each other in managing these conditions and to work together to maintain a healthy lifestyle through diet, exercise, and regular medical checkups.

By acknowledging and addressing age-related health issues in relationships, couples can deepen their bond, strengthen their communication, and find new ways to connect and experience love and passion in their 50s and beyond. Love truly knows no age, and with understanding, care, and creativity, intimacy can flourish at any stage of life. With understanding and compassion, couples can navigate these challenges together and continue to thrive in their relationship...

Handling Family Dynamics and Support Systems

As we age, our family dynamics and support systems play a crucial role in our emotional well-being and overall happiness. In your 60s and beyond, it is essential to navigate these relationships with care and understanding to ensure that they continue to bring positivity and support into your life.

One of the key aspects of handling family dynamics is setting boundaries. As we get older, it is common for family members to have different expectations and opinions about our lives. It is important to communicate openly and honestly with your loved ones about your needs and boundaries. This may mean setting limits on the amount of time you spend with certain family members or discussing topics that are off-limits.

Support systems are also vital as we age, especially when it comes to finding love and passion in our later years. Surrounding yourself with friends and loved ones who uplift and encourage you can make a world of difference in your pursuit of happiness. Whether it is joining a social group, attending community events, or simply spending quality time with those who make you feel good, having a strong support system can lead to a more fulfilling life.

Remember, it is never too late to find love and passion in your 60s and beyond. By nurturing your relationships with family and friends, setting boundaries, and building a strong support system, you can create a life filled with love, joy, and fulfillment. Embrace the journey and enjoy the ride.

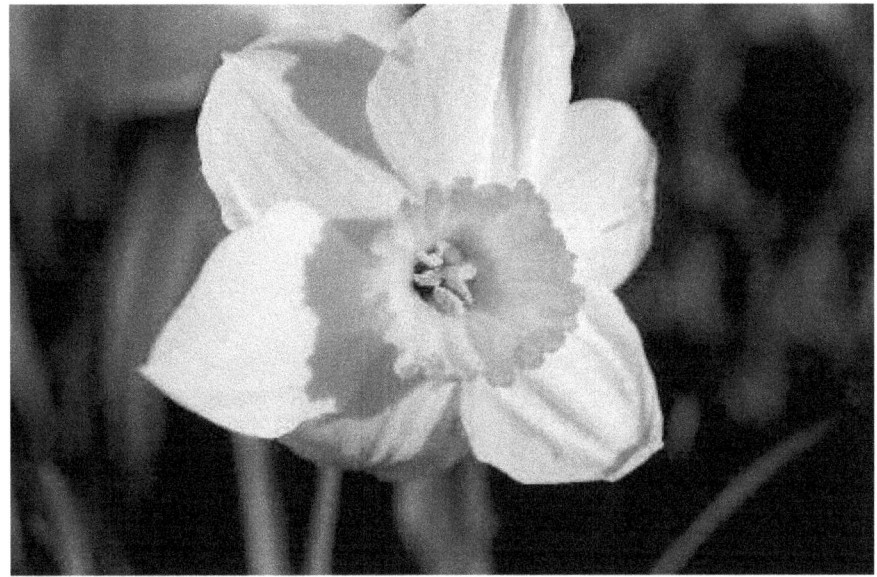

Celebrating Milestones and Achievements Together

As we reach our 50s and beyond, it is important to take the time to celebrate the milestones and achievements we have accomplished throughout our lives. Whether it is reaching a milestone birthday, celebrating a long and successful career, or achieving a personal goal, these moments are worth acknowledging and celebrating with our loved ones.

In the realm of love and passion, celebrating milestones and achievements together can strengthen our relationships and bring us closer to our partners. Whether it is celebrating a significant anniversary, reaching a relationship milestone, or simply expressing our love and gratitude for one another, these moments can help us rekindle the passion and love that brought us together in the first place.

One of the joys of growing older is having the opportunity to reflect on our lives and the journey that has brought us to where we are today. By celebrating our milestones and achievements together, we can share our stories, experiences, and wisdom with those around us. This not only helps us feel appreciated and valued but also allows us to connect with others on a deeper level.

By taking the time to acknowledge and celebrate our milestones and achievements together, we can create lasting memories and strengthen the bonds that tie us to our loved ones. So let us raise a glass, toast to our accomplishments, and continue to cherish the moments we have together, no matter what our age. Love knows no age, and neither should our celebrations of the milestones and achievements that define our lives.

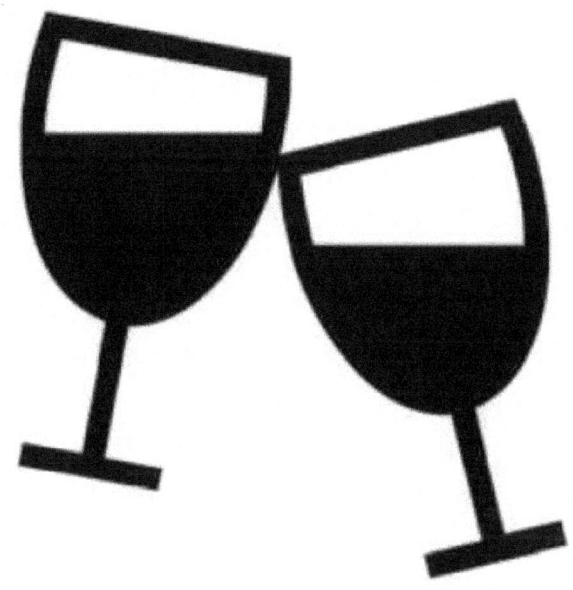

www.ingramcontent.com/pod-product-compliance
Lightning Source LLC
Chambersburg PA
CBHW051251120626
46547CB00014B/1899